Timothy Scott

The Ultimate Guide to Building Your Dream Body

Top 50 Exercises from Beginner to Advanced

Contents

1.

2.

3.

4.

5.

6.

Introduction

Welcome to *The Ultimate Guide to Building Your Dream Body: Top 50 Exercises from Beginner to Advanced.* Whether you're a newcomer to the world of fitness or a seasoned gym-goer looking to refine your workout routine, this book is your comprehensive road map to achieving a physique that reflects your strength, health, and confidence.

Building your dream body goes beyond mere aesthetics; it's about feeling empowered in your own skin, moving with agility, and having the endurance to tackle life's challenges head-on. Whether you want to sculpt lean muscle, increase strength, enhance flexibility, or improve overall fitness, this guide will equip you with the knowledge and tools to make tangible progress toward your goals.

In this book, I've curated the top 50 exercises across various difficulty levels, from beginner-friendly movements to advanced techniques used by professional athletes and fitness enthusiasts. Each exercise is carefully selected to target specific muscle groups, improve functional strength, and promote overall fitness.

Embark on this transformative journey with confidence and commitment. Whether you're starting from scratch or looking to refine your approach, *The Ultimate Guide to Building Your Dream Body* is your companion to achieving lasting results and embracing a lifestyle of strength, vitality, and well-being.

Let's begin your journey toward your dream body—one exercise, set, and rep at a time.

Chapter 1: Getting Started

Before you embark on your journey to build your dream body, it is crucial to define what that means for you. Setting clear and realistic goals will help you stay motivated and track your progress measurably and effectively.

Setting Realistic Expectations

Building your dream body will take time and dedication. Setting realistic expectations based on your current fitness level, lifestyle, and commitments is essential. Unrealistic goals can lead to frustration and a lack of motivation. Instead, aim for incremental progress and celebrate each milestone along the way.

Identifying Your Target Areas

Take time to identify which areas of your body you want to focus on. Whether it's sculpting your abs, building more muscular legs, or improving overall endurance, having specific goals will guide your exercise selection and training approach. Intense effort without the presence of intentional vision will get you nowhere.

Importance of Progressive Overload

Progressive overload is the principle of gradually increasing the stress placed upon the body during exercise to stimulate adaptation. This leads to gains in strength, muscle size, and endurance. Progressive overload can be achieved by increasing weight, repetitions, or intensity over time. Understanding and applying this principle will be vital in achieving your fitness goals.

1.2 Essential Equipment

Having the right equipment can significantly enhance your workout experience and effectiveness. Whether you're working out at home or in a gym, here are some essential items to consider:

Guide to Basic Gym Equipment

- **Dumbbells:** Versatile for upper body workouts and can also be used for lower body exercises.
- **Barbell and Plates:** Ideal for compound lifts like squats, deadlifts, and bench presses.
- **Resistance Bands:** Great for adding resistance to bodyweight exercises and mobility work.
- **Pull-Up Bar:** Essential for upper body strength development.
- **Yoga Mat:** Useful for floor exercises and stretching routines.

Alternatives for Home Workouts

If you prefer working out at home or don't have access to a gym, there are plenty of effective alternatives:

- **Bodyweight Exercises:** These can be done anywhere and are effective for building strength and endurance.
- **Resistance Bands:** Mimic the resistance of weights and can be used for various exercises.
- **Adjustable Dumbbells:** Compact and versatile, allowing for a range of weight options in one set.

Importance of Proper Footwear and Attire

Choosing the proper footwear and attire can enhance your performance and prevent injuries:

- **Shoes:** Invest in supportive shoes appropriate for your chosen activities (e.g., running shoes, cross-training shoes, lifting shoes).
- **Clothing:** Wear comfortable, moisture-wicking clothing that allows for freedom of movement.

1.3 Warm-Up and Stretching

A proper warm-up prepares your body for exercise by increasing blood flow to your muscles and raising your core temperature. It also helps reduce the risk of injury.

Dynamic vs. Static Stretching

- **Dynamic Stretching** involves moving parts of your body and gradually increasing reach, speed, or both through controlled movements. Examples include leg swings, arm circles, and torso twists.
- **Static Stretching** involves stretching a muscle to the point of mild discomfort and holding that position for a period of time (typically 15-30 seconds). Examples include quadriceps, hamstring, and lat stretches.

Importance of Warming Up

A good warm-up should last about 5-10 minutes and include movements that mimic the exercises you'll be doing in your workout. It prepares your muscles, joints, and cardiovascular system for the demands of exercise.

Sample Warm-Up Routines

- **Full Body Dynamic Warm-Up:** Include exercises like jumping jacks, high knees, bodyweight squats, and arm circles.

- **Specific Warm-Up for Resistance Training:** Before lifting weights, perform lighter sets of the exercise you're about to do, gradually increasing the weight.

By understanding your goals, equipping yourself properly, and warming up effectively, you'll set a solid foundation for your fitness journey. In the following chapters, we'll delve into the top 50 exercises that will help you build your dream body, starting with beginner-friendly movements and moving on to advanced techniques for those looking to challenge themselves further.

Chapter 2: Beginner Exercises

In this chapter, we'll explore foundational exercises perfect for beginners just starting their fitness journey. These exercises build strength, improve stability, and establish proper movement patterns. Whether you're working out at home or in a gym, mastering these fundamental movements will set the stage for more advanced workouts in the future.

2.1 Bodyweight Exercises

Before an aspiring fitness guru can take on the challenge of free weights, it is paramount to first master the weight of one's own body. The following exercises may seem impossibly simple, but dedication to the process will build a solid foundation for some of the more complex lifts found later in this chapter.

Push-Ups

Push-ups are a classic upper body exercise that strengthens the chest, shoulders, triceps, and core muscles.

- **Execution:** Start in a plank position with hands slightly wider than shoulder-width apart. Lower your body until your chest nearly touches the ground, then push back up to the starting position.
- **Variations:** Incline push-ups (using a bench or elevated surface), knee push-ups (on the knees for less resistance), and diamond push-ups (hands close together) to target different muscle groups.

Squats

Squats are essential for developing lower body strength, targeting the quadriceps, hamstrings, glutes, and core.

- **Execution:** Stand with feet shoulder-width apart, toes slightly turned out. Lower your body by bending your knees and hips, keeping your chest upright until your thighs are parallel to the ground. Push through your heels to return to a standing position.
- **Variations:** Bodyweight squats, goblet squats (holding a dumbbell or kettlebell at chest level), and split squats (one leg forward, one leg back) to vary intensity and challenge different muscle groups.

Planks

Planks effectively strengthen the core muscles, including the abdominals, obliques, and lower back.

- **Execution:** Start in a push-up position with elbows directly beneath your shoulders and forearms resting on the ground. Keep your body straight from head to heels, engaging your core muscles. Hold for as long as you can maintain proper form.
- **Variations:** Side planks (supporting yourself on one forearm and side of one foot), plank with shoulder taps (alternating touching each shoulder with opposite hand), and plank hip dips (rotating hips side to side) for added challenge.

Lunges

Lunges are excellent for targeting the quadriceps, hamstrings, and glutes and improving balance and coordination.

- **Execution:** Stand with feet hip-width apart. Step forward with one foot and lower your body until both knees are bent at a 90-degree angle. Push back to the starting position and repeat on the other leg.

- **Variations:** To engage different muscles and increase difficulty, perform reverse lunges (stepping backward instead of forward), walking lunges (alternating steps forward), and lateral lunges (stepping to the side).

Crunches

Crunches strengthen the abdominal muscles, particularly the rectus abdominis (six-pack muscles).

- **Execution:** Lie on your back with knees bent and feet flat on the ground. Place hands behind your head or across your chest. Lift your upper body off the ground by contracting your abdominal muscles, then lower back down with control.
- **Variations:** Bicycle crunches (alternating knee to elbow), reverse crunches (lifting hips off the ground), and leg raises (lifting legs while lying on your back) for targeting lower abs.

2.2 Dumbbell Exercises

Dumbbell Bench Press

The dumbbell bench press targets the chest, shoulders, and triceps and allows for a greater range of motion than a barbell bench press.

- **Execution:** Lie on a bench with dumbbells held directly above your chest, palms facing forward. Lower the dumbbells until your elbows are at 90 degrees, then press them back up to the starting position.
- **Variations:** Incline bench press (adjusting the bench angle for upper chest focus), decline bench press (adjusting the bench angle for lower chest focus), and neutral grip bench press (palms facing each other) for variation.

Dumbbell Rows

Dumbbell rows strengthen the upper back muscles, including the latissimus dorsi, rhomboids, and trapezius.

- **Execution:** Stand with a dumbbell in each hand, palms facing inward. Hinge forward at the hips, keeping your back flat. Pull the dumbbells towards your hips, squeezing your shoulder blades together, then lower with control.

- **Variations:** Single-arm dumbbell rows (one arm at a time), bent-over rows (using a bench for support), and renegade rows (from a plank position) for increased stability and core engagement.

Dumbbell Shoulder Press

The dumbbell shoulder press targets the deltoid muscles of the shoulders, as well as the triceps.

- **Execution:** Sit or stand with dumbbells held at shoulder height, palms facing forward. Press the dumbbells overhead until your arms are fully extended, then lower back down with control.
- **Variations:** Arnold press (rotating dumbbells during the press), seated shoulder press (using a bench for back support), and single-arm shoulder press (one arm at a time) to challenge shoulder stability.

Bicep Curls

Bicep curls isolate the biceps brachii muscles of the upper arm.

- **Execution:** Stand with dumbbells in hand, palms facing forward. Keeping your elbows close to your body, curl the dumbbells towards your shoulders, then lower back down with control.

- **Variations:** Hammer curls (palms facing each other), concentration curls (seated with elbow resting on thigh), and preacher curls (using a preacher bench) for targeting different parts of the biceps.

Tricep Extensions

Tricep extensions target the triceps brachii muscles at the back of the upper arm.

- **Execution:** Stand with dumbbell in hand overhead, palms facing inwards and arms fully extended. Bend at the elbows, lowering the dumbbell behind your head.

Dumbbell Shoulder Fly

The dumbbell shoulder fly targets the deltoid muscles of the shoulders, emphasizing lateral deltoids and overall shoulder stability.

- **Execution:** Stand with feet shoulder-width apart, holding a dumbbell in each hand at your sides, palms facing inward. Lift the dumbbells to the side until they reach shoulder height, keeping a slight bend in the elbows. Lower the dumbbells back down with control.

- **Variations:** Front dumbbell fly (lifting dumbbells in front of the body), rear deltoid fly (bending forward and lifting dumbbells behind the body), and bent-over dumbbell fly (bending at the hips and lifting dumbbells to the sides) for variation in shoulder muscle recruitment.

2.3 Machine Exercises

Leg Press

The leg press machine targets the quadriceps, hamstrings, and glutes, offering a safe and effective way to build lower body strength.

- **Execution:** Sit on the leg press machine with feet shoulder-width apart on the footplate. Push the weight away by extending your knees until legs are fully extended, then lower the weight back down with control.
- **Variations:** Narrow stance leg press (feet close together), wide stance leg press (feet wider apart), and single-leg press (one leg at a time) for added challenge and muscle isolation.

Lat Pulldown

The lat pulldown machine strengthens the latissimus dorsi muscles of the back, as well as the biceps.

- **Execution:** Sit on the lat pulldown machine with knees positioned under the pads. Grasp the bar with a wide grip, palms facing forward. Pull the bar down towards your chest, squeezing your shoulder blades together, then slowly release back to the starting position.
- **Variations:** Close grip pulldown (hands closer together), reverse grip pulldown (palms facing towards you), and single-arm pulldown (one arm at a time) to target different angles of the back muscles.

Leg Curl

The leg curl machine isolates the hamstrings at the back of the thigh.

- **Execution:** Lie face down on the leg curl machine with legs extended and the pad against your lower legs. Curl your legs towards your glutes by bending your knees, then lower back down with control.
- **Variations:** Seated leg curl (seated position with knees bent), single-leg curl (one leg at a time), and

stability ball hamstring curl (using a stability ball) for alternative hamstring exercises.

Chest Press Machine

The chest press machine targets the chest muscles (pectoralis major), shoulders, and triceps.

- **Execution:** Sit on the chest press machine with feet flat on the ground. Grasp the handles with palms facing forward. Push the handles away from your chest until arms are fully extended, then slowly bend your elbows to lower the handles back towards your chest.
- **Variations:** Incline chest press (adjusting seat angle for upper chest focus), decline chest press (adjusting seat angle for lower chest focus), and unilateral chest press (one arm at a time) for unilateral strength development.

Cable Row

The cable row machine strengthens the muscles of the upper back, including the rhomboids, trapezius, and rear deltoids.

- **Execution:** Sit on the cable row machine with knees slightly bent and feet placed on the footrests. Grasp the handle with palms facing each other. Pull the handle towards your abdomen, squeezing your shoulder blades together, then slowly release back to the starting position.

- **Variations:** Wide grip row (hands wider apart), narrow grip row (hands closer together), and single-arm cable row (one arm at a time) to target different parts of the back muscles.

Mastering these beginner-level exercises, whether using bodyweight, dumbbells, or machines, will lay a solid foundation for your fitness journey. Focus on maintaining proper form and gradually increasing the challenge as you build strength and confidence. In the following chapters, we'll delve into more advanced exercises to continue challenging your body and achieving your fitness goals.

Chapter 3: Intermediate Exercises

In this chapter, we'll explore intermediate-level exercises that build upon the foundational strength gained from beginner exercises. These movements incorporate more complexity, challenge coordination, and engage multiple muscle groups simultaneously. Whether you're looking to increase strength, improve muscular endurance, or enhance overall athleticism, these exercises will help you progress toward your fitness goals effectively.

3.1 Compound Movements

Deadlifts

Deadlifts are a compound exercise that targets the posterior chain muscles, including the hamstrings, glutes, lower back, and traps.

- **Execution:** Stand with feet hip-width apart, toes under the barbell. Bend at the hips and knees, keeping your back flat, and grasp the bar with an overhand grip. Lift the bar by extending your hips and knees until you are standing upright, then lower the bar back down with control.

- **Variations:** Sumo deadlift (wider stance), Romanian deadlift (focus on hamstring stretch), and trap bar deadlift (using a trap bar) for different emphasis and muscle engagement.

Barbell Squats

Barbell squats are essential for developing lower body strength, targeting the quadriceps, hamstrings, glutes, and core.

- **Execution:** Stand with feet shoulder-width apart, toes slightly turned out. Place the barbell across your upper back (behind the neck or on the traps). Lower your body by bending your knees and hips, keeping your chest upright until your thighs are parallel to the ground. Push through your heels to return to a standing position.
- **Variations:** For strength and stability, do front squats (barbell held in front of shoulders), overhead squats (barbell held overhead), and pause squats (pausing at the bottom position).

Bench Press

The bench press is a compound exercise that primarily targets the chest muscles (pectoralis major), shoulders, and triceps.

- **Execution:** Lie on a bench with feet flat on the ground and grasp the barbell with hands slightly wider than shoulder-width apart. Lower the barbell to your chest, keeping elbows tucked, then press it upward until your arms are fully extended. Lower the barbell back down with control.
- **Variations:** To vary muscle recruitment, you can do a close-grip bench press (hands closer together), an incline bench press (adjusting the bench angle for upper chest focus), or a decline bench press (adjusting the bench angle for lower chest focus).

Pull-Ups

Pull-ups are a bodyweight exercise that targets the back muscles (latissimus dorsi), biceps, and forearms.

- **Execution:** Grab a pull-up bar with palms facing away from you, hands slightly wider than shoulder-width apart. Hang freely with arms fully extended, then pull your body up until your chin is above the bar. Lower yourself back down with control.

- **Variations:** Chin-ups (palms facing towards you), weighted pull-ups (adding weight with a belt), and commando pull-ups (alternating grip) to challenge different aspects of back and arm strength.

Military Press

The military press (or overhead press) targets the deltoid muscles of the shoulders, triceps, and upper chest.

- **Execution:** Stand or sit with feet shoulder-width apart and grasp the barbell at shoulder height, palms facing forward. Press the barbell overhead until arms are fully extended, then lower it back to shoulder height with control.
- **Variations:** Push press (using legs to assist the press), dumbbell overhead press (using dumbbells for unilateral work), and Arnold press (rotating palms during the press) for variation in shoulder muscle recruitment.

3.2 Kettlebell Exercises

Kettlebell Swings

Kettlebell swings are dynamic exercises targeting the hips, glutes, hamstrings, and core muscles.

- **Execution:** Stand with feet shoulder-width apart and hold a kettlebell with both hands between legs. Hinge at the hips and swing the kettlebell forward, using hip thrust to propel it to chest height. Control the swing back down and repeat.
- **Variations:** For power and coordination, use single-arm kettlebell swings (one arm at a time), American kettlebell swings (overhead swing), and kettlebell snatch (swinging the kettlebell overhead in one motion).

Turkish Get-Up

The Turkish get-up is a full-body exercise that improves stability, mobility, and strength.

- **Execution:** Lie on your back with a kettlebell held in one hand, arm extended towards the ceiling. Roll onto your side and sit up while keeping the kettlebell overhead. Stand up while maintaining the kettlebell overhead, then reverse the movement to return to the starting position.

- **Variations:** Using a dumbbell instead of a kettlebell and breaking down the movement into stages to focus on technique.

Kettlebell Snatches

Kettlebell snatches are a powerful exercise that targets the shoulders, back, hips, and core.

- **Execution:** Stand with feet shoulder-width apart and hold a kettlebell in one hand between legs. Swing the kettlebell up and overhead in one fluid motion, using the hips and legs to drive the movement. Control the kettlebell back down and repeat.
- **Variations:** Single-arm kettlebell snatches (one arm at a time), high pulls (stopping the movement at chest height), and alternating snatches (switching arms with each rep) for coordination and power development.

Goblet Squats

Goblet squats are an effective variation of squats emphasizing core stability and lower body strength.

- **Execution:** Hold a kettlebell or dumbbell at chest height with both hands. Perform a squat by lowering your body until your thighs are parallel to the ground, keeping the weight close to your chest. Push through heels to return to standing position.
- **Variations:** For increased difficulty and balance, try pause goblet squats (pausing at the bottom position), sumo goblet squats (wider stance), and single-leg goblet squats (lifting one leg off the ground).

Kettlebell Rows

Kettlebell rows strengthen the upper back muscles, including the lats, rhomboids, and traps.

- **Execution:** Stand with feet hip-width apart, holding a kettlebell in one hand. Hinge forward at the hips while keeping your back flat. Pull the kettlebell towards your hip, squeezing your shoulder blade, then lower with control.
- **Variations:** For variations in muscle activation, try renegade rows (performed from a plank position),

alternating rows (switching arms with each rep), and high rows (pulling kettlebell towards chest).

3.3 Functional Training

Battle Ropes

Battle ropes are versatile for improving cardiovascular endurance, grip strength, and upper body power.

- **Execution:** Stand with feet shoulder-width apart and grasp the ends of the battle ropes. For different exercises, perform waves (alternating or simultaneous), slams (lifting and slamming ropes to the ground), and circles (making circles with the ropes).

Medicine Ball Slams

Medicine ball slams are a dynamic exercise that targets the entire body, focusing on power and explosive strength.

- **Execution:** Stand with feet shoulder-width apart, holding a medicine ball overhead. Slam the ball forcefully to the ground, bending at the hips and knees, then catch the ball on the rebound and repeat.
- **Variations:** Rotational slams (adding a twist to the slam), overhead slams (slamming the ball from

overhead), and partner slams (passing the ball back and forth) for variation.

TRX Suspension Training

TRX suspension training uses suspension straps to leverage bodyweight exercises for strength, stability, and flexibility.

- **Execution:** Adjust the TRX straps to desired length and perform exercises such as rows, push-ups, squats, and planks using the straps for added instability and resistance.
- **Variations:** TRX chest press (horizontal press movement), TRX single-leg squats (one leg supported by straps), and TRX atomic push-ups (bringing knees towards chest) for dynamic challenges.

Box Jumps

Box jumps are plyometric exercises that improve lower body power, explosiveness, and coordination.

- **Execution:** Stand facing a sturdy box or platform at knee height. Jump onto the box, landing softly with knees bent, then step or jump back down to starting position and repeat.

- **Variations:** Depth jumps (jumping off and immediately onto a higher box), lateral box jumps (jumping laterally onto the box), and single-leg box jumps (using one leg at a time) for progression and balance.

Agility Ladder Drills

Agility ladder drills enhance foot speed, coordination, and agility, making them ideal for athletes and fitness enthusiasts.

- **Execution:** Lay out an agility ladder on the ground and perform exercises such as high knees, lateral shuffles, crossover steps, and quick feet drills by stepping in and out of the ladder squares.
- **Variations:** Two feet in each square (quick feet), one foot in each square (single-leg drills), and lateral hops (hopping side to side over ladder) for variety in movement patterns.

Mastering these intermediate-level exercises will not only enhance your strength and endurance but also prepare you for more advanced challenges in your fitness journey. Focus on proper form, progression, and consistency to maximize your results. In the next chapter, we'll explore advanced exercises that will further push your limits and help you achieve your ultimate fitness goals.

Chapter 4: Advanced Exercises

Welcome to the realm of advanced exercises, where we push the boundaries of strength, endurance, and athleticism. These exercises are designed for individuals who have mastered the foundational and intermediate levels and are ready to take their fitness journey to the next level. From Olympic lifts to advanced bodyweight movements, each exercise challenges multiple muscle groups, enhances coordination, and boosts overall athletic performance.

4.1 Olympic Lifts

Clean and Jerk

The clean and jerk is a dynamic and explosive Olympic lift that targets the entire body, focusing on power, speed, and coordination.

- **Execution:** Start with a barbell on the ground, feet hip-width apart. Bend at the hips and knees to grasp the bar with an overhand grip. Explosively pull the barbell up to shoulder height (clean), then quickly dip under the bar and press it overhead (jerk). Lower the barbell back down with control.

- **Variations:** Hang clean and jerk (starting from the hang position), power clean (catching the barbell in a quarter squat), and split jerk (splitting legs to catch the barbell overhead) for technique refinement and power development.

Snatch

The snatch is another Olympic lift that improves explosive power, speed, and full-body coordination.

- **Execution:** Begin with a barbell on the ground, feet hip-width apart. Grip the bar with a wide overhand grip. Explosively pull the barbell up in one fluid motion, extending the hips, knees, and ankles while pulling yourself under the barbell to catch it overhead in a deep squat position. Stand up with the barbell overhead, then lower it back down with control.
- **Variations:** Hang snatch (starting from the hang position), power snatch (catching the barbell in a quarter squat), and snatch balance (developing speed and stability under the bar) for technical mastery and power development.

4.2 Plyometric Exercises

Depth Jumps

Depth jumps are advanced plyometric exercises that enhance reactive strength and explosive power.

- **Execution:** Stand on a sturdy box or platform at a moderate height. Step off the box and immediately upon landing, jump vertically or horizontally as explosively as possible. Land softly on the ground and absorb the impact with knees bent.
- **Variations:** Single-leg depth jumps (stepping off and jumping with one leg), lateral depth jumps (jumping laterally upon landing), and alternating depth jumps (jumping off and immediately into another jump).

4.3 Bodyweight Mastery

Muscle-Ups

The muscle-up combines a pull-up with a dip, showcasing upper body strength, coordination, and control.

- **Execution:** Start with hands on a pull-up bar, palms facing away from you. Perform a pull-up, then transition into a dip by pushing yourself above the bar until arms are fully extended. Lower yourself back down with control to complete one rep.

- **Variations:** Strict muscle-up (without kipping or swinging), false grip muscle-up (using a false grip on the bar), and weighted muscle-up (adding weight with a belt) for strength and skill development.

Handstand Push-Ups

Handstand push-ups develop upper body strength, shoulder stability, and balance.

- **Execution:** Start in a handstand position against a wall or freestanding. Lower your body until your head nearly touches the ground, then press back up to the starting position.
- **Variations:** Pike push-ups (with hips elevated), deficit handstand push-ups (using elevated platform for deeper range of motion), and freestanding handstand push-ups for advanced balance and strength.

One-Arm Push-Ups

One-arm push-ups are a challenging bodyweight exercise that targets the chest, shoulders, triceps, and core.

- **Execution:** Begin in a push-up position with feet wider apart for stability. Shift weight to one side and extend opposite arm straight out to the side or behind your back. Lower yourself towards the ground, then push back up to complete one rep.

- **Variations:** Archer push-ups (leaning to one side during the push-up), elevated one-arm push-ups (placing hand on an elevated surface), and weighted one-arm push-ups (adding weight with a plate or backpack) for progressive overload.

Clapping Push-Ups

Clapping push-ups are explosive push-up variations that improve upper body power and explosiveness.

- **Execution:** Perform a standard push-up, but explode off the ground forcefully enough to clap hands together before landing back in starting position.
- **Variations:** Plyometric push-ups (exploding off the ground without clapping), behind-the-back clap push-ups (clapping behind the back), and staggered clap push-ups (clapping hands while alternating arm positions) for dynamic upper body strength.

4.4 Advanced Core Exercises

Dragon Flags

Dragon flags are an advanced core exercise that targets the entire abdominal region and improves core strength and stability.

- **Execution:** Lie on a bench or mat with hands gripping the edge behind your head. Lift your legs and lower back off the ground, keeping your body straight. Lower your legs down slowly until they are almost parallel to the ground, then lift back up to starting position.
- **Variations:** Hanging dragon flags (using a pull-up bar for support), dragon flag negatives (focusing on the lowering phase), and dragon flag raises (lifting hips towards ceiling) for advanced core strength.

L-Sits

L-sits are an isometric exercise that targets the core, hip flexors, and shoulder stabilizers.

- **Execution:** Sit on the ground with hands placed on the ground next to hips. Lift your legs off the ground and extend them straight out in front of you, keeping them together and parallel to the ground. Hold this position with arms straight and shoulders engaged.

- **Variations:** Tuck L-sits (bending knees towards chest), L-sits on parallel bars (using parallel bars for support), and V-sits (lifting legs and torso to form a V shape) for advanced core control and stability.

Hanging Leg Raises

Hanging leg raises target the lower abs and hip flexors, improving core strength and stability.

- **Execution:** Hang from a pull-up bar with legs straight. Lift your legs towards the ceiling by flexing your hips and bending knees, keeping legs together. Lower legs back down with control to complete one rep.
- **Variations:** Toes-to-bar (lifting legs until toes touch the bar), windshield wipers (rotating legs side to side), and weighted hanging leg raises (adding ankle weights or holding a dumbbell between feet) for added challenge.

Ab Wheel Rollouts

Ab wheel rollouts are an advanced core exercise that strengthens the entire abdominal region and improves core stability.

- **Execution:** Kneel on the ground with hands gripping an ab wheel or barbell. Roll forward by extending your arms and torso, keeping abs tight and body straight, until arms are extended overhead. Roll back to starting position with control.
- **Variations:** Standing ab wheel rollouts (starting from standing position), kneeling ab wheel rollouts (kneeling on an exercise mat), and decline ab wheel rollouts (feet elevated on a bench) for increased difficulty and range of motion.

4.5 Advanced Functional Training

Ring Muscle-Ups

Ring muscle-ups are an advanced variation of the muscle-up performed on gymnastics rings, emphasizing stability and control.

- **Execution:** Start with hands on gymnastics rings, palms facing each other. Perform a pull-up and transition into a dip by pressing yourself above the rings until arms are fully extended. Lower yourself back down with control to complete one rep.

- **Variations:** False grip ring muscle-ups (using a false grip on the rings), strict ring muscle-ups (without kipping), and weighted ring muscle-ups (adding weight with a belt) for advanced ring strength.

Pistol Squats

Pistol squats are a challenging unilateral leg exercise that improves balance, flexibility, and lower body strength.

- **Execution:** Stand on one leg with the other leg extended straight in front of you. Lower your body into a squat position by bending your knee and lowering your hips towards the ground. Push through the heel of your standing foot to return to the starting position.
- **Variations:** Assisted pistol squats (using a support for balance), weighted pistol squats (holding a weight in front of you), and elevated pistol squats (using a platform under the extended leg) for progression and strength development.

Planche

The planche is an advanced gymnastic movement that requires significant upper body and core strength, as well as balance and stability.

- **Execution:** Begin in a push-up position with hands placed on the ground slightly wider than shoulder-width apart. Lean forward, lifting feet off the ground and straightening arms until body is parallel to the ground. Hold this position with arms fully extended and core engaged.
- **Variations:** Tuck planche (bending knees towards chest), straddle planche (spreading legs apart), and full planche (legs fully extended) for progression in planche training.

Front Lever

The front lever is a challenging gymnastic exercise that requires tremendous upper body and core strength, as well as body control.

- **Execution:** Hang from a bar with palms facing away from you, hands slightly wider than shoulder-width apart. Engage core and pull shoulder blades down while lifting legs until body is parallel to the ground.

Hold this position with arms fully extended and body straight.

- **Variations:** Advanced tuck front lever (bringing knees closer to chest), straddle front lever (spreading legs apart), and full front lever (legs fully extended) for progression and strength development.

4.6 Advanced Compound Variations

47. Jefferson Deadlift

The Jefferson deadlift, also known as the straddle lift, is an unconventional deadlift variation that challenges balance, strength, and coordination.

- **Execution:** Stand over the barbell with feet on either side of it in a wide stance. Grip the bar with one hand in front of the body and the other hand behind. Keeping a straight back, lift the bar by driving through the legs and hips. Lower the bar back down with control.
- **Variations:** Sumo Jefferson deadlift (wider stance), deficit Jefferson deadlift (standing on a platform), and single-arm Jefferson deadlift (lifting with one arm at a time) for variation in muscle recruitment and difficulty.

48. Hack Squat

The hack squat is a challenging leg exercise that targets the quadriceps, hamstrings, and glutes, emphasizing lower body strength and stability.

- **Execution:** Stand with feet hip-width apart and barbell behind your legs. Grip the barbell with hands behind you and lift it by extending through the hips and knees. Lower the barbell back down with control, keeping knees slightly bent throughout.
- **Variations:** Hack squat machine (using a hack squat machine for stability), front hack squat (gripping barbell in front of the body), and Bulgarian hack squat (elevating one leg on a platform) for additional challenge.

49. Sots Press

The Sots press is an advanced overhead press variation that improves shoulder stability, mobility, and overall upper body strength.

- **Execution:** Start with a barbell in a clean position at shoulder height. Lower into a deep squat, keeping elbows high and chest up. Press the barbell overhead while maintaining the deep squat position. Lower the barbell back down with control to complete one rep.

- **Variations:** Kettlebell Sots press (using kettlebells for added instability), dumbbell Sots press (using dumbbells for unilateral training), and seated Sots press (performing while seated) for different challenges.

50. Andersen Squat

The Andersen squat is a unique squat variation that challenges core stability and lower body strength.

- **Execution:** Begin with feet wider than shoulder-width apart and toes pointed outward. Hold a barbell behind the head, resting on the traps. Squat down as deeply as possible while keeping chest up and back straight. Push through the heels to return to standing position.
- **Variations:** Goblet Andersen squat (holding a kettlebell or dumbbell at chest level), Zercher Andersen squat (holding the barbell in the Zercher position), and overhead Andersen squat (pressing barbell overhead during the squat) for added complexity.

Congratulations on completing the advanced section of our journey to building your dream body! By now, you've delved deep into exercises that demand not only physical strength but also mental focus and discipline. Each exercise in this chapter has been carefully selected to push your limits, enhance your athleticism, and bring you closer to achieving your fitness goals.

Throughout these advanced exercises, you've challenged multiple muscle groups simultaneously, honed your coordination, improved your power output, and built the kind of strength that goes beyond just lifting weights. Whether you've conquered the explosive Olympic lifts, mastered the intricacies of bodyweight movements, or tackled the demanding core and functional exercises, each step has been a testament to your dedication and perseverance.

Remember, with great strength comes great responsibility—responsibility to listen to your body, to prioritize proper form and technique, and to approach each workout with intentionality. The advanced exercises you've learned are tools to be wielded thoughtfully, respecting the journey of physical transformation as a marathon, not a sprint.

As you integrate these advanced exercises into your training regimen, continue to set realistic goals, celebrate your progress, and stay committed to lifelong fitness. Whether your aim is to compete at an elite level, to surpass personal bests, or simply to maintain a healthy and strong body, the foundation you've laid here will serve you well.

In the final section of this book, we'll explore strategies for optimizing your training program, addressing common challenges, and ensuring sustainable progress towards your ultimate fitness aspirations. Keep pushing forward, stay motivated, and embrace the journey ahead with enthusiasm and determination. Your dream body awaits—let's make it a reality!

Chapter 5: Optimizing Your Training Program

$\mathbf{A}$s you embark on the advanced stages of your fitness journey, optimizing your training program becomes crucial for achieving sustained progress and reaching your ultimate fitness goals. This chapter explores key strategies that will help you maximize your workouts, prevent plateaus, and ensure long-term success.

Setting Clear Goals

Before diving into the specifics of your training program, it's important to establish clear and achievable goals. Setting Specific, Measurable, Achievable, Relevant, and Time-bound (SMART) goals gives you a clear roadmap and helps maintain focus and motivation throughout your fitness journey.

Designing an Effective Training Split

Choosing the right training split is essential for balancing workload and recovery. Whether you opt for an Upper/Lower split, Push/Pull/Legs split, or Full Body workouts, align your choice with your fitness goals, schedule, and recovery capacity.

Implementing Periodization Techniques

Periodization involves systematically varying intensity, volume, and exercise selection to optimize performance and prevent overtraining. Whether you prefer Linear, Reverse, or Undulating periodization, this approach helps continually challenge your body and maximize adaptation.

Embracing Progressive Overload

Progressive overload is the cornerstone of muscle and strength gains. Gradually increasing resistance, adding repetitions, reducing rest time between sets, and refining technique are all ways to ensure your muscles are consistently challenged and growing.

Prioritizing Recovery and Rest

Adequate recovery is essential for muscle repair and growth. This includes sufficient sleep, proper nutrition to support muscle recovery, active recovery activities like light stretching or yoga, and scheduled rest days to prevent burnout and reduce the risk of injury.

Nutrition and Hydration Strategies

Fuel your body with the nutrients it needs to support intense workouts and recovery. Pre-workout nutrition should include a balance of carbohydrates and protein, while post-workout meals or snacks should focus on protein to aid muscle repair. Staying hydrated throughout the day is also crucial for maintaining performance and overall health.

Monitoring Progress Effectively

Regularly tracking your progress is essential for staying on track and making necessary adjustments to your training program. This includes monitoring changes in body composition, strength gains, and overall workout performance. Use these metrics to gauge progress and adjust your approach as needed.

Overcoming Plateaus

Plateaus are a natural part of any fitness journey but can be overcome with strategic adjustments. Varying rep ranges, modifying exercises, incorporating deload weeks, and seeking guidance from fitness professionals can all help break through stagnant periods and continue making progress.

Sustaining Motivation Long-term

Maintaining motivation is key to sustaining long-term fitness success. Set short-term goals, celebrate achievements, find enjoyment in your workouts, and seek support from fitness communities or workout partners to stay motivated and committed to your fitness journey.

Embracing Long-term Sustainability

Finally, approach fitness as a lifelong journey rather than a short-term goal. Consistency, integrating fitness into your lifestyle, and cultivating a positive mindset towards fitness and health will ensure that your progress is sustainable and fulfilling over the long term.

By applying these principles and strategies, you'll optimize your training program to achieve lasting results and enjoy the journey towards a stronger, healthier you. Remember, each step you take brings you closer to your fitness goals, so stay committed, stay focused, and embrace the transformative power of your fitness journey.

Conclusion

Throughout this book, we've explored a comprehensive array of exercises, from beginner to advanced levels, designed to sculpt and strengthen your physique. Whether your goal is to gain muscle, shed fat, or improve overall fitness, you've gained valuable insights and tools to help you succeed.

From mastering foundational movements to tackling advanced exercises, you've learned the importance of consistency, proper technique, and listening to your body. Each chapter has been crafted to empower you with knowledge and practical steps to enhance your fitness journey.

As you move forward, remember that fitness is a lifelong commitment. It's about more than just physical appearance—it's about feeling strong, healthy, and confident in your own skin. Set SMART goals, stay consistent with your training, and embrace the process of continuous improvement.

Thank you for investing in yourself and taking steps towards a healthier, stronger you. Keep pushing your limits, stay motivated, and enjoy the rewards of your hard work. Here's to achieving and maintaining your dream body—let's continue this journey together!

If you found this book helpful, I'd be very appreciative if you left a favorable review for the book on Amazon.

www.ingramcontent.com/pod-product-compliance
Lightning Source LLC
Chambersburg PA
CBHW051707250726

48653CB00007B/2897